Low Carb

20+ Best Recipes and Weekly LCHF Meal Plan, LCHF Explained, Ketogenic Diet and Fat Adapted Training

Copyright 2016 by Dr. Dan Foss – All Rights Reserved

This document is geared towards providing exact and reliable information in regards to the topic and issue covered. The publication is sold with the idea that the publisher is not required to render accounting, officially permitted, or otherwise, qualified services. If advice is necessary, legal or professional, a practiced individual in the profession should be ordered.

- From a Declaration of Principles which was accepted and approved equally by a Committee of the American Bar Association and a Committee of Publishers and Associations.

In no way is it legal to reproduce, duplicate, or transmit any part of this document in either electronic means or in printed format. Recording of this publication is strictly prohibited and any storage of this document is not allowed unless with written permission from the publisher. All rights reserved.

The information provided herein is stated to be truthful and consistent, in that any liability, in terms of inattention or otherwise, by any usage or abuse of any policies, processes, or directions contained within is the solitary and utter responsibility of the recipient reader. Under no circumstances will any legal responsibility or blame be held against the publisher for any reparation, damages, or monetary loss due to the information herein, either directly or indirectly.

Respective authors own all copyrights not held by the publisher.

The information herein is offered for informational purposes solely, and is universal as so. The presentation of the information is without contract or any type of guarantee assurance.

The trademarks that are used are without any consent, and the publication of the trademark is without permission or backing by the trademark owner. All trademarks and brands within this book are for clarifying purposes only and are the owned by the owners themselves, not affiliated with this document.

Medical Disclaimer

You understand that any information as found within this book is for general educational and informational purposes only. You understand that such information is not intended nor otherwise implied to be medical advice.

You understand that such information is by no means complete or exhaustive, and that as a result, such information does not encompass all conditions, disorders, health-related issues, or respective treatments. You understand that you should always consult your physician or other healthcare provider to determine the appropriateness of this information for your own situation or should you have any questions regarding a medical condition or treatment plan.

You understand that the products and any related claims for such products have not been evaluated by the United States Food and Drug Administration (USFDA) and are not approved to diagnose, treat, cure or prevent disease. As such, you acknowledge that you are not relying in any fashion that the USFDA has approved of such products and claims.

You agree not to use any information on our book, including, but not limited to product descriptions, customer testimonials, etc. for the diagnosis and treatment of any health issue or for the prescription of any medication or treatment.

You acknowledge that all testimonials as found in our book are strictly the opinion of that person and any results such person may have achieved are solely individual in nature; your results may vary.

You understand that such information is based upon personal experience and is not a substitute for obtaining professional medical advice. You should always consult your physician or other healthcare provider before changing your diet or starting an exercise program.

In light of the forgoing, you understand and agree that we are not liable nor do we assume any liability for any information contained within this book as well as your reliance on it. In no event shall we be liable for direct, indirect, consequential, special, exemplary, or other damages related to your use of the information contained within our book.

This book offers health, fitness and nutritional information and is designed for informational and educational purposes only. You should not rely on this information as a substitute for, nor does it replace, professional medical advice, diagnosis, or treatment. Please discuss all medical and nutrition questions with your health care provider. If you have any concerns or questions about your health, you should always consult with a physician or other health-care professional.

The Food and Drug Administration have not evaluated the statements made within this book. The statements mentioned in this book are not intended to diagnose, treat, cure or prevent any disease.

Do not disregard, avoid or delay obtaining medical or health related advice from your health-care professional because of something you may have read in this book. The use of any information provided in this book is solely at your own risk.

Developments in medical research may impact the health, fitness and nutritional information that appear in this book. No assurance can be given that the information contained in this book will always include the most recent findings or developments with respect to the particular material.

The information provided by this book is believed to be accurate at the time it was created and it was based on research and our best judgment. However, like any printed material, information may become outdated over time. Information on this book may contain technical inaccuracies or typographical errors. Information may be changed or updated without notice.

All users agree that all access to and use of this book is at their own risk. This book or the author does not assume any liability for the information contained herein, be it direct, indirect, consequential, special, exemplary, or other damages; including intangible losses, resulting from: (i) the use or the inability to use our book, our services, or any services or products of any third party; or (ii) statements or conduct of any third party.

If you are in the United States and think you are having a medical or health emergency, call your health care professional, or 911, immediately.

Table of Contents

Medical Disclaimer iii

Introduction vii

Chapter 1: About the LCHF Diet.. 8

Chapter 2: The Ketogenic Food Pyramid 13

Chapter 3: What to Eat and not Eat 17

Chapter 4: Mistakes with the LCHF Diet 24

Chapter 5: Ketogenic and Fat-Adapted Training 28

Chapter 6: The Grocery Guide to Ketosis 35

Chapter 7: Twenty Great LCHF Recipes............................ 40

Chapter 8: A Nutritional Plan for LCHF 59

Conclusion... 63

Other Books By This Author 64

About the Author 65

Introduction

Thank you for taking the time to download this book: Low Carb High Fat 101: 20+ Best Recipes and Weekly LCHF Meal Plan, LCHF Explained, Ketogenic Diet and Fat Adapted Training.

This book covers the topic of the Low Carb High Fat Diet, and will teach you everything you need to know about the LCHF diet.

At the completion of this book you will have a good understanding of how the LCHF diet works and also some great meals and tips that can be used to help you reach your goals.

Once again, thanks for downloading this book, I hope you find it to be helpful!

Chapter 1: About the LCHF Diet

You might be wondering what the LCHF diet is and how do you get started. Well, this chapter will go into the ins and outs of this diet, what it stands for, and some of the nuances of this sort of diet. There is quite a bit of information here, and this chapter will give you everything that you need to know about this remarkable diet.

What is the LCHF diet?

Well, it's essentially that you don't eat a ton of carbs, but instead, you eat a lot of fat.

The typical American diet has a ton of carbs in it. Carbs, while you do need them, shouldn't be taken within excess, but, if you look at your diet, you probably take about ten times the amount that you actually need every single day. That's why many people keep the fat that's on their body; they pump themselves full of carbs 24/7.

Fat has gotten allot of negative press over the last few years with many people. It's been seen as evil because people think fat is what makes you fat. But the reality is it's not. Carbs are really not as necessary as people think, but fat keeps you fuller, allows you to burn off the excess weight on your body, and in general, is allot more nutritionally dense. Plus, you're helping your body instead of damaging it.

In essence, the low-carb high-fat diet is a lifestyle change to help your body become more efficient at burning fat and help your body to function in a correct manner. By the time you finish this book, you'll see what it entails for an individual, and why it's important to understand all ins and outs. For some people, this diet might seem hard, but at the end of the day, it's not so bad.

Science Behind LCHF

You might also be wondering if there is any science behind this sort of diet. Well there is, and its possible to lose allot of weight on this diet. It's especially useful for those with heart disease and diabetes. Over the last ten years more and more research has been done on the LCHF diet. A recent study has showed those on a low carb high-fat diet reduced their risk for type 2 diabetes. All of study participants were overweight, on cholesterol drugs, and had heart disease. One of the first studies done on this diet was in 1955 when James Hayes MD a cardiologist was curious to see if the LCHF diet increased bad cholesterol or LDL levels. He took 23 of his obese heart disease patients and put them on a LCHF diet over a 6-week period. In conclusion although his patients remained on statin drugs to lower cholesterol something amazing happened, at the end of the 6-week period their average weight loss was 5.2% of their body weight and their cholesterol stayed steady but there triglyceride level lowered.

On average, those that follow this diet actually lose about 5% of their body fat after six weeks alone, which means that from this diet alone, a person who weighs 200 pounds can definitely lose at least 10 pounds.

What's incredible is research is showing that this diet has no detrimental effects on cholesterol levels, but instead, is boosting the good cholesterol.

There are also reports of atherosclerotic plaque being removed from a person's arteries, which is the cause of cardiovascular diseases and stroke. Blood serum glucose and insulin levels also lowered which helped those that were pre-diabetic literally stop sugar handling problems in their tracks. There are tons of studies being done on this, and many types low-carb high-fat diets came about because of this, such as Atkins, and also Weightwatchers. When you get started with LCHF you need to follow it very closely, but if you do, it's been scientifically proven to help you lose weight.

Dangers of LCHF

While this diet is great in some ways for improving the health of the body, there are a few dangers to this as well. You should be really watching these if you feel you are trying to reach ketosis or a ketogenic state.

Ketosis is defined as the production of what are called ketone bodies which come from the metabolism of fat. When your burning more fat for fuel you are in a ketogenic or as I call a fat adapted state. Although there are a ton of health these are some of the things to watch out for.

The first is poor gut health. If you have poor gut health to start with, it can often cause a lot of issues for you with the LCHF diet. You'll have to repair your gut health with allot of vegetables and some probiotics as well as eating a lot of fat and not a ton of carbs. Eating fermented vegetables such as kimchi and sauerkraut can help your gut flora. Also supplementing with kombucha, a fermented tea with live bacterial cultures. If you do have a poor or leaky gut you can also try supplementing with glutamine powder. We'll discuss this more at a later time.

Often on this diet, if your goal is ketosis, you will need to make sure that you don't let your carbs exceed 50 grams. If it does, then it will be much harder for you to get through this, so be smart when you're on this diet, and watch out for excessive intake of carbs.

If you eat a lot of fat and protein already and eat limited fruits and vegetables, while you do get an increase in lean muscle mass, you might also start to develop chronic inflammation in the body. This can come from the number of free radicals that can form from the increase in consumption of animal products. For many people, if you consume very little fruits and vegetables, you can have a lower antioxidant capacity, and often, this is a deficiency in many who have a low carb high protein diet. You can take a supplemental water soluble vitamins which help to boost the antioxidant capacity of the body. The water-soluble vitamins are Vitamin A, C, and E or the ACE vitamins.

Another thing to watch out for is bowel movements. With high fat and especially high protein diets your digestion can slow down and you could become constipated. A great fix for this is to make sure that you're also eating a lot of vegetables and other food items with fiber as well.

Obviously, before you get onto this type of diet, you must consult your doctor. Do this before you begin so you can reduce the risk of anything, which might come about as a result of the diet.

What are the Benefits of LCHF?

There are, in fact, tons of health benefits for the LCHF diet, and there are many great things that can come from utilizing it and making it part of your lifestyle.

For starters, when you're on the LCHF diet, you'll be able to lose weight. You will be eating less, but feeling full, and your insulin levels won't spike and then crash like they normally do. This will result in decreased insulin resistance.

You will not have the feeling of hunger as often due to the increase in quality foods you are consuming and you will also feel fuller for a longer period of time.

You will also be having more nutrient-dense foods. Many of these fatty foods are full of great vitamins and minerals, which will lead you on a path to better health in the future while on this diet.

Along with this too, you'll also start to notice that fat in trouble areas, such as your stomach, is starting to go away, replaced with a body that looks good, and feels great. Visceral fat is the fat that surrounds your organs and it spells disaster for your body if its in high amounts. Once you start getting into ketosis with the LCHF diet you will really start to see a reduction in the visceral fat and this can have a major impact on your health. Remember it's not so much how we feel but how we heal.

Overall, when you do the LCHF diet, you will be able to really improve your life, making it better, more enjoyable, and less sickness and disease. If you ever feel like you want to get rid of the negative toxins in the body, go LCHF, for it has been proven to reduce heart disease and a whole slew of other health issues.

The LCHF diet is great for those looking to improve their body in numerous ways. The next chapters will show you just how it is done, what you can do to better yourself, and the various elements that are associated with LCHF.

Chapter 2: The Ketogenic Food Pyramid

The Ketogenic food pyramid is pretty easy to understand. There are three main elements that you should be worried about with this diet, and you should start to look at this before you begin.

Fat

Fat is typically what you are adding in large amounts when you're working with the ketogenic and LCHF diet. The ketogenic diet mainly relies on this, so you should make sure that when you're working with this sort of diet, you should have about **75%** of your diet be fat.

Fat should be saturated and unsaturated fat, but make sure that the saturated fat isn't man-made fat such as processed meats in lunchmeats or genetically modified (GMO). Make sure that the saturated fats are natural, for they will help your body get into ketosis, so you will be able to do much better with the action of burning fat.

When you get into the ketogenic or fat adapted state is when you really start to see the results. You'll be eating allot of fat, and almost no carbs, so you should start to realize just how much fat you'll be having when you're on this sort of lifestyle diet.

As a general rule if you're consuming 2,000 calories you should consume approximately 56-78 grams of fat. I know this seems like allot of fat but there are some great tricks to do this so stay with me.

Protein

Protein is the next largest part of this pyramid, and it accounts for about 20% of what you're going to have every single day. Proteins are typically found in the fats such as lean meats and vegetables. Protein is what helps you to build muscle. However, one big element of protein, which many of us seem to forget, is that when we have it we don't get enough fiber, which will result in digestive issues and inflammation. When you're looking to start on this diet, you should monitor your fiber intake as well so that it can help you with understanding the diet that you're about to take on. The best sources of low carb fiber are flax and chia seeds.

Protein is something that you should be watching for in your diet. Many of us, when we are doing this sort of diet, will rely on proteins that are often very simple such as protein powders. You should go primarily with a lot of nutrient-dense proteins such as those found in cage free, free range, and grass fed animal meats and not manufactured proteins, because often, those sorts of proteins will start to become harder to digest. With allot of the manufactured proteins comes artificial sweeteners, additives, preservatives, and sometimes simple sugar and carbs. Be smart about the type of protein that you consume and keep it as organic and fresh as possible.

As a general rule keep your protein intake between .8-1.2grams per kilogram. The higher end if you are more physically active.

Carbohydrates

Oh, carbs. They get a bad name on the ketogenic diet, and on the LCHF diet, but you shouldn't go cold turkey with them altogether. Some starches are good for you, such as those in some low glycemic fruits and vegetables, and sometimes, you might start to have these as well. When you're engaging in the ketogenic diet, you should look at how much carbs you're taking in. It shouldn't exceed 50 grams, which is the equivalent of only a few slices of white bread (and yes I'm recommending that you avoid bread and gluten all together). Anything over 50-100 grams you might still lose weight but you won't be in ketosis. Going in the 50-100 grams range is a great maintenance to continue to lose 1-2 pounds per week without going into ketosis where you will shed pounds faster.

As a rule try to avoid processed or refined carbs. Basically if you walk into a supermarket it is everything on the shelves in the center. Often, these are filled with substances that are essentially a substitute for the actual low-carb items that you've had in the past. For many of us, there are a lot of times when we might believe that's the right choice at the right time, but it's not. Those types of carbs aren't good for your body at all, so its best to avoid them. These refined and processed carbs are the killers: obesity, weight gain, skin disorders, and many diet related diseases including heart disease, hypertension, insulin resistance, type 2 diabetes, and some cancers.

However, you should go for carbs in very small amounts. Don't overeat carbs, which is often the issue when starting this diet. You should start with this diet by getting rid of any high-carb junk foods that you have in your home. This can be anything from candy bars to potato chips, flour and corn tortillas, fruit juices, vinegar products, GMO products, soy products, grains and rice, and factory farmed foods. These types of foods you should avoid. Watch them carefully, because you can ruin your ketosis if that's what you're going for. So be mindful, make sure that you do keep up with everything when you are doing this.

With the ketogenic food pyramid, you'll start to realize over time that it's pretty easy to do, to engage in, to try, and by the end of this, you'll be able to have the lifestyle and health you deserve. Be smart with everything, start to understand just what you're doing, and keep in mind these three components to your diet. These are the three core areas of not only the ketogenic diet, but also the LCHF diet, so do be smart with this, and make sure you know what you're getting into when choosing what to eat.

Chapter 3: What to Eat and not Eat

You've probably wondered just what you should be eating and what you shouldn't be eating. Well, this chapter will tell you everything you need to know on that. This chapter will describe what it is you should avoid when you are engaging in the ketogenic diet or an LCHF diet, and what you can do to make it even better.

What to Eliminate

This is probably the toughest part of the diet. Choosing what to eliminate in terms of foods is an individual process. When it comes to carbs, not all of them are created equal. Some are complex carbs, which are good in small amounts, and some are bad and simple, such as junk food.

However, there are some foods that you will learn right away to eliminate, and that's where this section comes in.

The first is junk foods, candy, or anything processed. This includes processed snacks. These are loaded with a ton of carbs, and if you ever want to see just how damaging they are, look at the nutrition facts on these. You'll see just how many carbs are present in just one serving. All too often, that's about the equivalent of what you should be having every single day. Not a pretty sight, so step away from doing that.

You should also start to get rid of any grains that aren't whole grains and replace them with low-carb grains. I also recommend looking at the label and if it has gluten in it or is produced in a factory that contains gluten don't take it. Many low-carb grains are either made yourself with psyllium husk powder or chia/flax seeds, or you can find them in the health food store. But if bread and pasta are your favorites, you might be in for quite a rude awakening when you start this diet, because those are going to have to go. The time to go gluten free is now!

With fruits and vegetables, some of them are okay. Low-carb fruits and veggies are allowed, but with some of the higher carb ones, such as legumes, various sugary fruits, potatoes, and the like, they're very starchy, and that's actually something you want to aim to avoid. When you're engaging in this diet, learn about what sorts of carbs each of these fruits have, and start to eliminate them accordingly, so that you're not stuck trying to scramble and keep them out of your sight. Here is an easy formula (although there are exceptions) to help you with fruits and veggies. The majority of fruits are high in sugar or what is called high-glycemic. So for fruits the higher up they are in the air, the more sugar they contain, as they are closer to the sun. For vegetables the lower in the ground the more sugar they contain, as they have more roots which store more sugar.

When it comes to alcohol of any forms, it should be taken out of the diet. It's not that alcohol is bad in small amounts, it's that it has got a ridiculous amount of calories and carbs. Take a look at a serving of a six-pack of beer, all the carbs that are riddled in there. It's not something that you need, so it's best if you do take the time to eliminate those from your diet as well. If you do have to have alcohol I recommend going for the lowest sugar content wine, which is red wine. Pinot Grigio is a favorite and 5 oz has less than 1 gram of sugar.

Finally, if you see any of those low carb alternatives at the store, you should eliminate those too. Like I mentioned before stay as natural as possible. Avoid the zero carb drinks and artificial sweeteners, preservatives, and additives. They don't work, and often, they're not what you should start to look for, so instead, start to keep everything in order for your body by only having those low-carb foods that you know are good, and start to have more fats. Again my goal is to get your healthier inside and out.

Loading Up on Fats

You're probably wondering just what you can eat now that you're not able to have carbs. You might be scrambling wondering just what in the world you can have. Well, what about fats? There is a load of fats out there, and you can indulge in these to a strong degree.

Trans fats should be avoided. Trans fats are industrial fats and are typically synthetic and used in many processed goods that are packed. These are typically the baked goods and vegetable oils that you see. You're already probably eliminating these, but make sure that you do take the time to remove them from your diet further as well. In fact in 2015 the Food and Drug Administration (FDA) has set a 3-year plan to remove trans fats from the market. Trans fats have been proven time and time again to raise our LDL's and lower or HDL's. It's a wonder why they are still on our shelves in the supermarket.

However, when it comes to fats, there are so many that you can eat that will go a long way. For example, lean meats such as fish and chicken are great, and they're highly encouraged. Fatty fruits such as avocados and coconut (technically not a fruit) are also encouraged on this sort of diet, so make sure you have a wealth of those. Any healthy fat is good. You should also look into flavoring up these fatty foods as well. They taste good, but a common complaint with many people who do this, is that they get sick of how much meat or veggies there are in this, and often they get bored of the foods. However, if you start to liven it up with these various spices, it'll make these fatty foods taste better.

Eggs are great to use on this diet. Eggs are full of healthy fats and vitamins, and they also have a lot of protein as well. I recommend getting free range and cage free egg's as much as possible. When it comes to cooking with certain oils, there are also other fats you can have as well. Olive oil is one of them, and it's one of the best oils to have when you're cooking. It's healthy, full of unsaturated fat, and it is an excellent means to not only cook with but also as a garnish. If you can find it look for real olive oil such as this one here. If you do not wish to use olive oil, sesame oil, flaxseed oil, and especially coconut oil work great.

Coconut oil is the best of the bunch. It is a saturated fat, but it's a very healthy saturated fat with so many benefits to it. With coconut oil, you get a whole wealth of vitamins, minerals, and the like, and often, with many people, it can be the best one to cook with. Start to incorporate coconut oil into your diet today, and your body will thank you. This by far has been my best way to get more fat into my diet. Later on in this book I'm going to go over more LCHF recipes but I want to share my favorite one here, its called ketogenic fat bombs. Here is the recipe:

Keto Bombs

Ingredients:

- 1 cup organic virgin coconut oil
- 1 cup organic peanut butter or almond butter
- 4 Tablespoons (1/4 cup) raw cacao powder
- 2-3 drops of Stevia or Cinnamon liquid

Directions:

- Melt the Coconut in a pot over low heat
- Add the Peanut Butter and Cacao
- Add the Stevia or Cinnamon
- Wait for everything to melt, avoid boiling
- Pour into a glass measuring cup or Pyrex
- Pour into cupcake tray and place in the freezer

Wait about an hour and enjoy with Whip Cream! Yum!

Calories: 145

Fat: 15 grams

Carbs: 2 grams

Along with this, however, is coconut in general. Coconut has so many great health benefits, and it tastes great too. Coconut has strong antibacterial, antiviral, and antifungal properties. If you have yeast issues in or on your body coconut will work wonders for it along with the LCHF diet. There's even coconut milk and water, which is full of fats and other vitamins. When it comes to loading up on fats, coconut is one of the true ways to go, because not only can you eat it, but there's a ton of other great benefits as well.

Keeping up with the Proteins

Proteins are your final element to work with. With proteins, you'll be able to build muscle in the body. However, with protein, there is also the factor of making sure that you have enough fiber in the diet. Proteins are necessary for this sort of diet, but there is also the factor of you need to make sure that you also get adequate fiber to help with the digestion. Otherwise, you'll give yourself stomach irritation inflammation, and the like. When you're working on the LCHF diet, you should make sure that proteins are your key part in it, and make sure that if you do need to add more fiber, you incorporate some low carb veggies in order to do this.

Important proteins are typically found in meats. However, some nuts, while some are filled with carbs, others are actually filled with proteins and healthy fat. Here is an example of these: almonds, macadamias, walnuts, cashews, and red skinned peanuts. You should have these as a snack, and make sure that your fat intake coincides with everything else.

Another great source of protein is fish and fowl. You should make sure it's not riddled with saturated fat or trans fat, but often, you get a chunk of your protein from this. Again look for organic and wild caught.

Dairy, such as milk, cheese, and cream can sometimes be filled with carbs if it's processed. However, natural, organic cheese and specialty cheese have less of this issue, and if you're looking for a good, wholesome cheese that works for you, this is often one of the best. Plus, there is much you can do in order to get this together, and you can have these proteins right at your disposal. Try them, and you'll be able to incorporate so much more into your diet than you've ever expected. Add a little heavy cream onto your fat bombs for added taste.

With this chapter, you've seen some of the various parts of what to eat and not eat. This is a guide to what you should be watching for, and what you should grab, so make sure you keep these in mind when you're shopping, for it'll make your life that much easier.

Chapter 4: Mistakes with the LCHF Diet

With the LCHF diet, there are a few mistakes that one can make. These are typically pretty easy to rectify, but they should be known, because often, this is something that many people don't watch out for. This chapter, however, will give you a right sort of mindset on what kinds of mistakes you can make with this diet, and how you can rectify them.

The first is eating too many carbs. This is often the issue that many of us suffer from. This is something that you should be mindful of, and you should watch for this in your diet. If you start to see that your carb intake is too high despite fixing it up by lowering some carbs, seek to lower it further. This can be anything from cutting out any cheat foods, to even getting rid of high sugar fruits that you might have. Your goal is to eliminate as many carbs as possible, and that's what this diet will do for you. Remember if you are doing intense exercise either aerobic or anaerobic exercise you should raise your carbs a little bit but not too much. Exercising fasted with no carbs and on a high fat diet is proving scientifically to be one of the best things you can do for performance, health, and longevity.

Along with this, another major mistake people make, is that they will not eat any vegetables. However, vegetables are very important. The reason for this is because they are filled with so many types of fiber, so you should make sure that you include them in your diet. Fiber will allow you to digest various elements in your diet, and when you're dealing with a lot of fat and proteins, you're going to need it. However, you also need fruits and vegetables because of the vitamin and mineral content. Make sure to stick to low glycemic fruits and vegetables that are low in sugar. Fruits and vegetables are loaded with essential vitamins and minerals and it's imperative that you make sure you do have these for your body. If you don't you'll end up having more issues than you would care to want to have. Many times we focus on just the fats, but you need other vitamins as well.

Another mistake is not enough protein. You're going to need lots of fat to keep yourself full and to help spend energy, but you need protein as well to build muscle. If you're losing all that fat on your body, you're going to want to tighten it up and make sure you maintain your lean muscle mass. That's the purpose of this getting enough protein. You should make sure that you don't overdo it per se, but you should also make sure that you don't just let yourself go because you don't have any.

You should also get rid of the mistake of having frequent cheat days. Cheat days are important maybe once a week but not all the time. There are many low-carb desserts out there that you can have, so make sure that you don't have anything that's riddled with carbs. The reason for that is because if you do that sort of thing, you're going to end up cheating more, and that's a big mistake many of us do make. So don't jeopardize your body and your results.

Finally, you should always consult your doctor before getting into this. That is very important, because often, the problem with many who start on the LCHF diet is that they don't medical clearance. This leads them onto the path of they need to do this, but then they realize they're putting their health at risk, and overall, that's just not smart. Make sure you have medical clearance before you do something of that sort. An important aspect of this is making sure you are working with a doctor that understands health and nutrition. Many doctor's will look at the amount of fat you are taking an be quick to put you on a statin drug to lower your cholesterol or tell you to stop the LCHF diet all together. The reality is most medical doctor's have little to no training in nutrition.

An important aspect of this diet is Cholesterol. A common mistake people make is looking at cholesterol one dimensionally. HDL cholesterol is commonly know as good cholesterol and a high fat diet will typically increase your HDLs. Triglycerides will typically be lowered with a high fat diet. The issue for people is the LDL cholesterol and when they discuss LDLs with their doctor or see that they are high this will cause some alarm. What you need to know is this, there is new research concerning LDLs. Recent research has shown that LDLs can be measured in two ways. One called LDL-C measuring the concentration of cholesterol carried by LDLs in the blood, and the second LDL-P measuring the number LDL particles in the blood. What's of interest is the size of the LDL particles. Current research has shown that its LDL particle size is far more precise of an indicator for cardiovascular disease (CVD) than total LDL cholesterol count. Therefore the larger the LDL particles the less health risk for CVD a person has.

Confused yet? Basically, eating more fat can raise your cholesterol but also raises the size of your LDL particles. Is that good for me? Current research is pointing to the benefits of high fat diets for Alzheimer's, Dementias, and many more neurological disorders. The take away is that our Brain is 60% fat and you are what you eat.

When you're engaging in the LCHF diet, make sure you keep these in mind. The last thing you want to do is hurt your body, and this chapter went over some of the great things you can watch out for when engaging in this diet. It's a great way to lose weight and build a better body, but just make sure you're doing it right so you're not hurting yourself and others.

Chapter 5: Ketogenic and Fat-Adapted Training

You might be wondering if there is any sort of physical training you can do with this. There is and this chapter will go over three great methods that you can look at when you're attempting to train your body. I'm a firm believer in any change that its 80% diet and 20% exercise.

Exercise Fuel Tanks

In our body we typically have two fuel tanks: glycogen or sugar and fat or adipose tissue.

Our muscles and liver carry approximately 2,000 calories of glycogen or sugar. Have you ever skipped a meal, or skipped eating for a day and were surprised that you still had energy? That was the glycogen fueling you throughout the day. The fact is our body needs sugar and it's the only way we can produce energy, which in biochemistry terms is called ATP (Adenosine Triphosphate). What happens is the liver has to convert the proteins, carbohydrates, and fats that we eat into glucose. The problem comes when we eat too much sugar its too easy for our body to convert it to energy and as easily as its converted to energy the quicker it is gone. Think of this tank as kindling on a fire. When you start a fire you use small branches and leaves, which burn very quickly. Glycogen or sugar does exactly that it burns quickly and then it's gone. Do you we need this fuel tank? Yes! But lets talk about the other tank.

The second tank we have is fat or adipose tissue. Most of us carry at least 10-20 pounds of extra body weight and sometimes much more. Lets face the facts even if we are super skinny we still have fat. Our fat tank was built for one reason, protection. When we eat excess sugar and our blood glucose levels rise too high our liver becomes taxed signals the body that we need to store that sugar for a future date, thus we have visceral fat that surrounds our organs and subcutaneous fat that is just below our skin. Which ones more dangerous? It's actually the visceral fat or as many call stubborn fat which has the most detrimental effect on our health. On average we have 40,000 calories of fat stored in our body at any given time. Imagine if our body was adapted to burn that fat for fuel instead of burning sugar. Think of this tank as a nuclear reactor. Maybe not on an atomic level but just imagine the amount of energy we could generate from 40,000 calories or more stored in our body.

So which tank is best? Well it depends on what we want to do. If we need quick energy then of course we need glycogen and we have more than enough in our body than the need to consume more. If we need sustained energy then using the fat stores would be the best way to keep us going for a lifetime. Renewable and sustained energy sources, time to stop playing with kindling and put some real logs on the fire.

Maffetone Method

Dr. Phil Maffetone developed the Maffetone Method as a way to help endurance athletes become more fat adapted or keto-adapted in a ketogenic state. Essentially, this type of exercise focuses on fat-burning activities and ways you can really train an aerobic system. In this training system, you're looking to work with making sure that you do work to stimulate the slow-twitch fibers, which will improve the heart and lungs, boost the circulation, and enhance the brain function. This formula will allow you to look for what is called your MAF Heart Rate, allowing you to effectively keep it at that level so that one can work with the fat-burning system.

A great way to see if you're burning more fat and becoming more fat adapted is to train with a heart rate monitor. This can be done with any aerobic training such as running, cycling, swimming, or any other aerobic endurance sport. Essentially when you are at a lower heart rate you are burning more fat for fuel and when you are at a higher heart rate you are burning more sugar for fuel.

The first step is getting a heart rate watch. I don't recommend any particular brand but great starter watches at the time of this writing are the Polar M400 found here and the Garmin Fenix 3 found here.

The next step is determining your optimal heart rate zone for maximum fat loss and to really get you keto-adapted or in a fat adapted state. Dr. Maffetone has done a tremendous amount of work in this field and you can read his paper on the subject here but I'm going to give you a quick guide. Make sure you read his paper as there are a few exceptions to the rule when doing this calculation. Basically what you do is take 180BPM and subtract your age. Then if you are just getting started with heart rate training subtract 5 more which gives you what he calls your MAF HR or your Maffetone HR. Then subtract 10 to give you the range that you want to exercise in. Here is an example:

1. If you are 50 years old this would be 180-50 or 130BPM

2. Then subtract 5 if you are just getting started so 130-5 is 125BPM

3. Then your MAF HR would be 125 – 10 or between 115 to 125BPM

I recommend programming your watch manually to either beep at you when you go below your MAF HR or when you go above. As in this example set your watch to beep below 115BPM or above 125BPM. Now when you go above or below make sure that you either slow down or walk if running or cycling to get your heart rate back into the MAF HR zone.

Keep you heart rate in this zone and remember that heart rate training takes time. Slow and steady is the motto. Two things are going to happen. The first is that you will start to build your aerobic capacity or basically the amount of oxygen in milliliters that you can use in one minute/kg of body weight. Basically that means that a higher aerobic capacity equals more work that you can do at the same heart rate. All this is happening because your body is more fat adapted and ketogenically adapted to burn more fat for fuel. There are a number of things that affect aerobic capacity such as heart size and strength, concentration of hemoglobin in your blood, density of your capillaries, and density of mitochondria in your cells. Mitochondria are the powerhouses of our cells that burn sugar for fuel so when you build those levels up you can burn fat and fuel more efficiently. When you are more fat adapted you are actually changing the physiology of your body to burn more adipose tissue for fuel thus getting you hooked directly into that nuclear reactor that we call the fat tank.

What does this mean for athletic performance aerobically? Essentially this is making you not only a more efficient athlete but a healthier one.

Will you get faster? Yes! Will you shed body fat? Yes! But remember heart rate training and fat adaptation is not an overnight thing and will take time. In the beginning if you are running in your MAF HR zone and move out of it you will have to stop and walk allot and I mean allot. As you become more fat adapted and boost your aerobic capacity you will not only shed pounds of fat but go faster, farther, and harder than ever. With this sort of training, you're provided with the means to effectively and easily train yourself for success.

As a general rule keep 80% of your training aerobic to burn more fat.

Interval or Burst Training

Another way to enhance the amount of fat that you do burn is interval or burst training. You should, in this sort of instance, start going at one speed for a bit, and then you burst to a higher speed for a certain period of time. This is one of the means to burn fat on the body. The reason for this is that when you are running at a slower pace you are burning more fat, then when you kick into the faster interval you are burning more sugar with the goal of burning off more of your muscle glycogen.

To do this, you choose how long you're going to run at a certain speed. Say it's about five minutes of an easy pace, and two of a very hard pace. The hard pace is essentially a sprint, and you maintain that through all of this. Do that, and then you go straight back to that, and soon, you'll notice that it gets harder as you increase the number of intervals. You should have a stopwatch to tell you when you should be going easy, but from there, you can determine the number of sets to do. Ideally, doing about 20 minutes of these sets if the best one, and it's certainly what will work when it comes to improving the interval training that you have.

As a general rule keep 20% of your training anaerobic to burn more fat.

Intermittent Fasting 16/8

Intermittent fasting is a great protocol and strategy to implement in LCHF diets and also incorporating fasted exercise. Intermittent fasting might seem like a strange sort of means to actually eat, but in truth, it is one of the best ways for those that are looking to build muscle but minimize fat. In some cases, you will gain muscle and lose fat. Many use this, and it's one of the best ketogenic training methods.

What this means is simple. You will fast for about 16 hours each day, and then, in the 8 hours of each day, you eat what you need. You should eat what you normally would, and it doesn't have to be scheduled. Many people will fast overnight, and from there, they will skip breakfast and have lunch and their first meal during the early afternoon.

For breakfast you can have water, tea, or coffee and if you exercise during your fasted state you can have branch chain amino acid's (BCAAs) up to 30 grams a day.

With this type of fasting, you'll be eating a lot of high-fat foods with low carbs. The concept behind intermittent fasting is that you are eating fatty foods to help you keep fuller for longer. If you just ate carbs during this time, you also won't be able to do this. The amount that you eat is your typical amount of these 8 hours so that you will eat your full calorie limit then. After that, you fast, and it's actually one of the best ways to lose fat.

It's really the best one if you don't' feel like wanting to work with heart monitors and such. If you do this, all you got to do is dictate a time, have a meal plan, and then go from there.

With these types of training, you can build muscle while still losing fat, and you'll be able to do so effectively, and to a result, while engaging in the low-carb high-fat lifestyle.

Chapter 6: The Grocery Guide to Ketosis

When you're thinking about the types of foods you can eat while on the ketogenic diet, or even when you're just putting together an LCHF lifestyle, there are a few things to keep in mind. This chapter will give you an excellent grocery guide to what you want.

- Vegetables: always get some low-carb veggies. These are high in nutrients, and some of them are also high in fats. You can find these in the produce section. Remember the leafy greens and vegetables closer to the ground will contain less sugar.

- Lean meats: make sure you get some of these while you're at the store. These are what will typically be your nightly proteins or whenever you have lunch or dinner. Make sure you go for organic and grass fed as much as possible.

- Eggs, milk, and another high-fat dairy: get these, without any of that "low-fat" stuff to it, because if it's low in fat, it's which in carbs. Make sure that you try to get organic when possible as well. Make sure you go for organic and cage free or free range and grass fed as much as possible.

- Fruits: only get a few fruits, and stay away from ones that are typically high in sugars and carbs. Look for organic fruits and remember the ones lower on the vine or lower to the ground typically have lower sugar content.

- Grains: when getting grains, look for whole grains and grains that aren't' processed. Avoid white bread and manufactured breads at all costs. You can create your low-carb alternatives. My advice go gluten free so skip grains.

- Spices and herbs: these will be your food's best friends. Getting some of these to put on your meals and then eating them is essential, so make sure that you do this. Look for organic and those that have no additives or preservatives.

- Bacon and other meats: Enjoy them but remember have a little moderation. Don't eat a ton of red meat, and don't have a ton of high saturated fat meats. You should make sure that you avoid processed meats and go organic, grass-fed meats if you're getting beef. You should try to substitute them for leaner meats, such as bison instead of beef if you want to make burgers.

- Nuts: some nuts are great, others are high in carbs. Almonds and walnuts are certainly right. You should stay away from those mainstream pre-packaged nuts such as planters unless of course, they don't contain a ton of carbs. Often, however, they throw a lot of preservatives in there that you don't obviously need.

- Coffee: coffee with butter and coconut put in there every day is actually an amazing meal alternative. You can get these at the store, and you can create this sort of coffee every single morning. Putting butter in there allows the coffee to have fat, and coconut gives it both fat and flavoring. It's a great breakfast sort of supplement, and it'll keep you full during the day if you're looking for something that's an alternative.

- Baked goods; any and all baked goods should be crossed off your grocery list. The only exception is if you're getting some items to create some low-carb desserts, which are there, but you'll have to make them yourself.

- Anything "low carb": these should also be avoided like the plague. The reason for this is because they're often not something that'll help you, and they're typically something that you should watch out for too. They also have replacement preservatives in this that can mess with ketosis.

- Locations: when shopping, avoid the inner aisles and stick around the outer aisles. Typically the healthier stuff is put on the outside, and the unhealthy stuff is inside.

- Knowing this, you will be able to achieve an LCHF lifestyle in no time, and very easily as well.

Getting started with a Ketogenic Diet can be overwhelming. When I first got started I was confused as to what I could buy and what I couldn't buy.

So I created this shopping list. Of course there are things that might not be on the list that you can find. This is just a good list to get started.

Most of my non-perishable item's I purchase online thru Amazon Prime.

I included the links below for Amazon to the non-perishable items. Use this as a guide:

Here is a great Shopping List to get you started with Ketogenic Diets:

Non-perishable items: (many available on Amazon)

Almonds

Macadamia Nuts

Extra Virgin Olive Oil

Unrefined Organic Coconut Oil

Avocado Oil

MCT Oil

Stevia Liquid

Cinnamon Liquid

Coconut Flour

Almond Butter

Peanut Butter

Almond Flour

Sesame Oil

Ghee

Cacao Powder

Chicken Bullion

Coconut Milk

Bison Bars - Epic Brand

Organic Coffee

Grass Fed Protein Powder

Perishable Items: (look for organic, grass fed, cage free as much as possible)

Grass-fed beef
Wild salmon
Chicken thighs
Low Carb Veggies
- Cauliflower
- Zucchini
- Celery
- Onion

- Cabbage
- Bell Peppers
- Squash
- Spinach
- Romaine lettuce

Shredded and hard cheeses
Avocado
Sour Cream
Heavy Cream
Butter
Eggs
Salami / Prosciutto
Herbs and spices
Broth: Chicken and Beef
Coffee (Organic)
Olives

Chapter 7: Twenty Great LCHF Recipes

Now that you know all about the LCHF diet, it's time to go over 20 easy, delicious recipes to help cater to this diet that is perfect for you.

Cheesy Roll-Ups

Ingredients:

- 12 slices of cheese of choice

- 12 slices of butter

- Seasoning of choice

Directions:

- Put the cheese on cutting board. Put butter in cheese slicer and slice it thin

- Put the butter on top of cheese and then roll up. Can be served as a snack

Calories: 200

Fat: 20 grams

Carbs: 2 grams

Cheesy Chicken Breasts

Ingredients:

- 4 chicken breasts

- 1 pepper

- 2 Tbs pickled jalapenos, chopped

- Salt and pepper for taste

- 1 cup shredded cheese

- 2 Tbs olive oil

- 1 garlic clove

- ½ tsp cumin

- 3 oz. cream cheese

- 4 toothpicks

Directions:

- Preheat oven to 350
- Chop and sauté the garlic and peppers. Let cool
- Put the jalapenos, cheese, and spices, mixing
- Cut lengthwise through the chicken to open it
- Put cheese batter in there and close it with the toothpicks
- Season, fry it with oil, put it in a baking dish
- Put the rest of the cheese batter on top and let cook for 15 minutes until thoroughly cooked

Calories: 350

Fat: 22 grams

Carbs: 8 grams

Eggs on the Go

Ingredients:

- 12 eggs

- Filling if you want such as olives, feta, or herbs

- Salt and pepper for taste

Directions:

- Preheat oven to 400
- Put cupcake liners in there, put an egg in each form and add filling. Season to taste, then bake for 15 minutes or until cooked

Calories: 150

Fat: 10 grams

Carbs: 3 grams

Parmesan Roasted Green Beans

Ingredients:

- 1 egg

- 1 tsp onion powder

- 2 pinches pepper

- ½ cup grated Parmesan cheese

- 2 Tbs olive oil

- ½ tsp salt

- 1-pound green beans

Directions:

- Preheat oven to 450

- Put eggs, oil, and spices into a bowl. Put beans in there and stir until beans are covered

- Remove extra liquid and mix in Parmesan cheese

- Put it on baking sheet and bake for 15-20 minutes

Calories: 170

Fat: 13 grams

Carbs: 3 grams

Keto Quesadillas

Ingredients:

- 6 low-carb tortillas

- 1 oz. leafy greens

- 1 tsp olive oil

- ½ pound shredded cheese

- Lettuce or spinach

Directions;

- Put the tortillas on a cutting board

- Put half cheese into there, then some leafy greens, and then put the rest of cheese and the tortillas

- Heat a frying pan with oil. Roast it for about a minute until the bread is a nice color and cheese is melted

- Divide and serve immediately

Calories: 400

Fat: 20 grams

Carbs: 4 grams

Stuffed Mini Bell Pepper

Ingredients:

- ½ pound mini bell peppers

- 1 oz. chorizo

- 2 Tbs olive oil

- ½ pound cream cheese

- 1 tsp mild chipotle sauce

- 1 Tbs cilantro

Directions:

- Slice peppers into half lengthwise and remove core

- Chop up the sausage and herbs, then mix in the cheese, oil, and spices into a bowl, then adding in the rest of the ingredients

- Put it onto the bell peppers, and then serve it

Calories: 200

Fat: 15 grams

Carbs: 5 grams

Oven Paprika with Rutabaga

Ingredients:

- 2 pounds chicken, thighs or drumsticks

- 4 oz. olive oil

- Salt and paper for taste

- 2 pounds root celery

- 1 Tbs paprika powder

- 1-cup mayonnaise if desired

Directions:

- Preheat oven to 400 and split chicken into quarters
- Peel rutabaga and then cut into 2-inch pieces
- Salt and pepper to taste and put the pepper and chipotle on top
- Add in the olive oil and mix
- Bake this for about 40 minutes or so and lower heat towards the end of the time
- Serve with mayonnaise

Calories: 320

Fat: 18 grams

Carbs: 3 grams

Cheese Chips

Ingredients:

- ½ pound sliced cheese

- ½ tsp paprika powder

Directions:

- Preheat oven to 400 and then put cheese slices on baking sheet

- Put paprika on top and bake for about 8-10 minutes.

- Look towards end to see that slices don't' burn or have a bitter taste

- Serve with guacamole

Calories: 200

Fat: 10 grams

Carbs: 2 grams

Oven Baked Brie

Ingredients:

- 9 oz., Brie

- 1 garlic clove

- Rosemary or thyme

- Salt and pepper

- 2 oz. nuts of choice

- 1 Tbs herbs

- 1 Tbs olive oil

Directions:

- Preheat oven to 400 and put cheese on baking sheet with parchment paper
- Chop nuts and garlic, mix with rest of ingredients, seasoning to taste
- Put nut mix on cheese and bake for 10 minutes until it's a nice color. Serve lukewarm

Calories: 150

Fat: 8 grams

Carbs: 1 gram

Hollandaise Sauce

Ingredients:

- 4 egg yolks

- 10 oz., butter

- 3 Tbs squeezed lemon juice

- Salt and pepper

Directions:

- Crack eggs and put it in bowl, keeping egg whites
- Melt butter, but don't let it brown
- Beat butter one drop at a time until it's increased until it's a thick sauce. Continue until all butter is added. The white milk protein at the bottom of pan shouldn't be included
- Put lemon, salt, and pepper to taste, stirring before serving with some veggies

Calories: 120

Fat: 10 grams

Carbs: 2 grams

Rotisserie Chicken with Béarnaise Sauce

Ingredients:

- 2 rotisserie chickens

- Some leafy greens of choice

Béarnaise sauce:

- 4 egg yolks

- 2 pinches onion powder

- 2 tsp tomato paste

- Salt and pepper for taste

- 2 t white wine vinegar

- 1 chili, chopped and deseeded

- 8 oz. butter

Directions:

- Cut chicken in half and make salad with greens on another dish
- Crack open eggs and separate from yolks, mixing in the vinegar, chili, and onion powder
- Whisk in a drop of butter at a time until it thickens and is added. Don't include the white milk protein
- Add in vinegar and tomato paste, putting in the salt and pepper to taste. Keep it warm in double broiler
- Fry the chicken and serve with a salad that you made before

Calories: 430

Fat: 22 grams

Carbs: 6 grams

Keto lasagna

Ingredients:

- 2 Tbs olive oil

- 1 onion

- ½ cup tomato paste

- 1 tsp salt

- ½ cup water

- 1-pound ground beef

- 1 garlic clove

- ½ tsp dried basil

- ½ tsp ground black pepper

Cheese topping

- 2 cups sour cream

- ½ cup grated Parmesan cheese

- ¼ tsp ground black pepper

- 1 cup shredded cheese

- ½ tsp salt

- ½ cup fresh chopped parsley

Directions:

- Make pasta sauce the day before
- Peel and chop onions and garlic and fry them. Put in ground beef and fry till golden. Put in tomato paste and spices
- Stir with water, let boil, lower heat and then let it cook for 15 minutes
- Preheat oven and put the sour cream with cheese, except for 2 T for topping. Add in salt and pepper and stir parsley
- Put lasagna and the sauce in layers of a baking dish
- Put sour cream and batter with rest of Parmesan on top

- Bake for 30 minutes or until lasagna has surfaced. Serve with salad

Calories: 450

Fat: 22 grams

Carbs: 5 grams

Caprese Snack

Ingredients:

- ½ pound cherry tomatoes

- 2 Tbs green pesto

- ½ pound mini mozzarella cheese balls

- Salt and pepper to taste

Directions:

- Slice the tomatoes and mozzarella in half. Put in pesto and stir
- Serve with seasoning to taste

Calories: 140

Gat: 9 grams

Carbs: 2 grams

Chocolate Mousse

Ingredients:

- 2 cans coconut milk

- 1 tsp vanilla extract

- 2 tsp cocoa powder

- 1 t honey

Directions:

- Let coconut milk sit in fridge for at least 4 hours

- Open can and scoop out the thick cream. Save coconut water

- Whisk in cream, honey, and vanilla for a couple of minutes. Add cocoa powder and whisk more

- Serve in dessert bowls

Calories: 220

Fat: 8 grams

Carbs: 4 grams

Spicy Nuts

Ingredients:

- ½ pound nuts of choice

- 1 Tbs olive oil

- 1 tsp paprika or chili powder

- 1 tsp salt

- 1 tsp cumin

Directions:

- Mix all ingredients in frying pan on medium temperature until warmed
- Let cool and then serve

Calories: 200

Fat: 10 grams

Carbs: 4 grams

Low Carb Casserole

Ingredients:

- 1 rotisserie chicken

- ½ pound diced bacon

- 2 cups heavy whipping cream

- 1 tsp yellow curry powder

- 1 banana

- 2 Tbs butter

- ½ pound mushrooms

- 3 Tbs chili sauce

- Salt and pepper for taste

- 3 T salted peanuts

Directions:

- Preheat oven to 400

- Cut mushrooms into small pieces and fry with bacon and butter

- Season to taste and cut and debone chicken

- Put chicken pieces in bacon dish with the bacon and mushrooms. Add the banana

- Whisk in the whipping cream and then put in chili sauce, curry, and the salt and pepper over to chicken

- Bake for 20 minutes and put some chopped peanuts on top before serving

Calories: 450

Fat: 25 grams

Carbs: 9 grams

Mozzarella Stuffed Meatballs

Ingredients:

- 2 pounds ground beef
- 1 Tsp salt
- 2 Tbs water
- Butter for frying
- 1 Tbs dried basil
- 2 pinches pepper
- 4 oz., mozzarella cheese

Directions:

- Put the ground beef in a bowl, adding spices and water and mix with hands or a fork
- Form 10 patties about 4 inches in diameter
- Cut mozzarella into 10 pieces and put one on each patty. Close into ball
- Fry in butter until juices clear and the meat shrinks

Calories: 220

Fat: 12 grams

Carbs: 4 grams

Low-carb Garlic Bread

Ingredients:

- 2 Cups almond flour
- 2 Tsp baking powder
- 2 Tsp apple cider vinegar
- 3 egg whites
- 5 Tbs psyllium husk powder
- 1 Tsp sea salt
- 2 cups boiling water

Garlic butter:

- 4 oz., grass fed butter at room temp

- ½ Tsp garlic powder

- ½ Tbs salt

- 2 Tbs chopped parsley

Directions:

- Preheat oven to 350 and mix the dry ingredients
- Boil water and put vinegar and egg whites together to whisk
- Form 10 pieces and roll hot dog bun style
- Bake for 40-50 minutes
- Mix in garlic butter while baking by mixing all ingredients and chilling them.
- When done, let the buns cool and then get the garlic butter. Cut them in half and put the garlic butter on top
- Turn oven to 425 and bake it for about 10-15 minutes until golden brown

Calories: 300

Fat: 18 grams

Carbs: 5 grams

Low Carb Seed Crackers

Ingredients:

- ½ cup almond flour, pumpkin seeds, sunflower seeds, flax seeds, and sesame seeds

- 1 Tsp salt

- 1 cup boiling water

- 1 Tbs psyllium husk powder

- ¼ cup melted coconut oil

- Sea salt

Directions:

- Preheat oven to 300 and mix all dry ingredients before adding water and oil
- Put dough on a baking sheet, seasoning with sea salt
- Bake on a rack for 45 minutes, checking occasionally. Let dry for another 15 minutes
- Turn off oven and let dry. Break into pieces and cover with butter

Calories: 110

Fat: 10 grams

Carbs: 3 grams

Keto pancakes

Ingredients:

- 6 eggs
- ¾ cup coconut milk
- 1 pinch salt
- Butter or coconut oil
- ½ cup coconut flour
- 2 Tbs melted coconut oil
- 1 tsp baking powder

Directions:

- Move yolk from egg whites and whisk the egg whites with salt, using a hand mixer

- Whisk until stiff peaks form and put aside

- Put together egg yolk, coconut milk, and oil in another bowl

- Add in flour and baking powder

- Fold the egg whites into batter, let sit for about 5 minutes

- Fry them for a minute on each side and then serve with butter and berries with some whipped cream. Yum!

Calories: 330

Fat: 14 grams

Carbs: 6 grams

These 20 recipes will help you get started with the LCHF diet easily. They're simple, effective, and so good for you as well.

Chapter 8: A Nutritional Plan for LCHF

With many people, getting on the LCHF diet is quite hard. However, there are many ways to make this easier on you. This chapter will go over some nutritional plans to help you get through a week of the LCHF diet

Day one:

- Breakfast: Omelet with mixed veggies, frying them in coconut oil

- Lunch: Yogurt with blueberries and almonds. Can also have a wrapped cheese in butter

- Snack: Fat bombs, Nuts/Seeds

- Dinner: Lettuce wrapped cheeseburger with veggies and salsa

Day 2:

- Breakfast: Bacon with eggs and bulletproof coffee with coconut oil

- Lunch: Burgers that are left over with veggies

- Snack: Fat bombs, Nuts/Seeds

- Dinner: Buttered salmon and veggies

Day 3:

- Breakfast: Eggs and vegetables fried in coconut oil

- Lunch: Shrimp salad with olive oil

- Snack: Fat bombs, Nuts/Seeds

- Dinner: Grilled chicken with veggies

Day 4:

- Breakfast: Simple omelet with vegetables

- Lunch: Coconut milk smoothie with almonds, berries, and some kale

- Snack: Fat bombs, Nuts/Seeds

- Dinner: Steak and veggies

Day 5:

- Breakfast: Bulletproof coffee with coconut and butter

- Lunch: Chicken salad with olive oil dressing

- Snack: Fat bombs, Nuts/Seeds

- Dinner: Grass-fed pork chops with leafy greens

Day 6:

- Breakfast: Paleo pancakes

- Lunch: Mixed veggies in hollandaise sauce and a smoothie

- Snack: Fat bombs, Nuts/Seeds

- Dinner: Bison burgers lettuce wrapped with leafy greens

Day 7:

- Breakfast: Bacon and eggs, or keto pancakes

- Lunch: Keto quesadilla with a salad

- Snack: Fat bombs, Nuts/Seeds

- Dinner: Fish grilled with veggies and butter

This meal plan can always be substituted out with some of the various recipes that were given to you in the earlier chapter. As you can see, some were incorporated, but if you're not super great in the kitchen, you can always substitute them out.

For a snack, which is sometimes included if you have a longer span of eating, I suggest going back to the previous chapter and finding one that best fits you. Look for ones that are fitting, and from there, make them before you go out. I always recommend fat bombs as a great snack throughout the day. Also nuts and seeds are a great snack just remember they do have some carbs so don't go overboard.

If you do work outside of the home, which many people do, there is a way to incorporate these various foods into it. You should start by making sure you have a meal plan in place every single day, and you should also take the time to ensure that you do follow it. If you have to make multiple foods, make them the night before, and from there, you can put them in little Tupperware containers and bring them with you to your work. If there is a microwave you can heat it, but if not, just bring some salads and food that won't' spoil. You can do this with dinners as well by preparing them ahead of time and going from there.

If you do need a dessert for whatever reason, the previous chapter had some desserts and snacks. Try them, and see how they go. You can also find other low-carb desserts out there too, so you're not fully denying yourself all of this.

This chapter went over some of the great elements you can have in terms of meal plans for your LCHF diet. You should have a more thorough understanding of this type of diet, and from there, you'll be able to improve over time and create the best meals that you possibly can, no matter what happens to you next.

Conclusion

Thank you again for taking the time to check out this book.

Going low carb and high fat is often something that many of us struggle to do, but with this book, you were able to see just how possible it is, and how you'll be able to truly make sure that you have everything squared away for this. The LCHF lifestyle is quite a bit of a struggle for some, but by the end of this, you should be able to see just what sort of impact you have with this, and how to get into this diet.

With that being said, it's time for the next step. Your next step is simple but effective, and the next step is to start getting on the LCHF diet. You should start changing up your diet to incorporate a low-carb lifestyle, and you should make sure that you do have this all in place before you begin. Consult a doctor before you begin, and make sure that you know what you're doing. You deserve to yourself to have the best and healthiest lifestyle possible, and that's how this diet will benefit you.

If you enjoyed this book, please take the time to leave me a review on Amazon. I appreciate your honest feedback, and it really helps me to continue producing high quality books.

Please, leave a review, or check out my website www.fatadapteddoc.com .

Other Books By This Author

I hope you enjoyed reading this book! I have put allot of work into studying and researching Intermittent Fasting, Ketogenic Diets, Low Carb High Fat Lifestyles, Fat Adaptation, and Heart Rate Training.

I have some other books that I have written on Amazon that I think you might be interested in. Below is a list of my other books, along with direct links to their pages on Amazon.

Intermittent Fasting: 6 effective methods to lose weight, build muscle, increase your metabolism, get ketogenic, and get healthy

Ketogenic Diet Plan: 30 Day Meal Plan, 50 Ketogenic Fat Burning Recipes for Rapid Weight Loss and Unstoppable Energy

Low Carb High Fat 101: 20+ Best Recipes and Weekly LCHF Meal Plan, LCHF Explained, Ketogenic Diet and Fat Adapted Training

About the Author

Dr. Dan Foss graduated from Western States Chiropractic College in 2003. His fresh outlook on health, nutrition, and exercise has helped thousands of people not only get well but stay well for a lifetime. His goal as a Chiropractor is to help educate and empower people to understand how the human body works so that they can make the best decisions regarding their health and well-being. Over the last 13 years he has practiced Chiropractic and the last 7 years has owned and operated Pura Vida Chiropractic, a wellness center based in San Antonio, Texas. When not practicing he is a father, husband, coach, mentor, and amateur endurance athlete. Currently he is training for his first 50K ultra marathon in the mountains of Big Bend National Park.

Printed in Great Britain
by Amazon